HOW-TO

ALDARA USAGE

How Imiquimod Helps Your Body Fight Skin Conditions and Stimulates Healing

Dr. Tim Cahill

Contents

CHAPTER ONE 3
   Introduction 3
   How Aldara (Imiquimod) Works 7
   Therapeutic Uses of Aldara 13

CHAPTER TWO 28
   Application and Usage 28
   Side Effects of Aldara 36
   Precautions and Contraindications 45
   Drug Interactions and Resistance 52
   Conclusion 56

THE END 63

CHAPTER ONE

Introduction

Aldara or, in its generic form, imiquimod, is a topical cream mainly indicated for the treatment of skin disorders like actinic keratosis, superficial basal cell carcinoma, and genital warts. Unlike conventional drugs that act directly on the symptoms or the invading organism, Aldara elicits an immune response from the body to combat the disease and thus stands as a class apart from the other modes of treatment. This immunomodulatory property sets it apart from other topical agents and extends its versatile role in dermatology. This manual will cover how

Aldara works, its therapeutic uses, methods of applications, side effects, and things to consider clinically.

How Aldara (Imiquimod) Works

Imiquimod is a drug classified as an immune response modifier. It does not have a specific mechanism of action that attacks viruses or tumor cells directly but rather gives an impulse to the immune system of the body to act against abnormal cells or viral infections. This is achieved by initiating the innate immune system to increase the expression of cytokines, such as interferonα, interleukin6, and TNFα.

Principal Mechanism: Activation of Toll Like Receptor 7 (TLR7):

Imiquimod binds to TLR7 on immune cells, thereby inducing the secretion of cytokines. These signaling molecules facilitate the recruitment of immune cells, including macrophages and natural killer cells, to the site of application, thus potentiating the capacity of the host to resist infection or malignant cell proliferation.

Antiviral and Antitumor Activity: While stimulating the immune response, Aldara helps not only in eradicating viral infections but also in destroying precancerous or cancerous cells.

That's the beauty of an immunomodulatory mechanism: the immune response is taught in the long run to recognize and destroy similar insults in the future.

Therapeutic Uses of Aldara

Because Aldara can modulate the immune system, it has a wide range of clinical applications. The most effective applications of Aldara occur with skin conditions that have an infectious or cancerous component.

1. Genital and Perianal Warts (Caused by HPV)

One of the most common uses of Aldara includes the treatment of external genital and perianal warts caused by human papillomavirus (HPV). These warts may be rather difficult to treat with traditional methods, such as cryotherapy, and recurrence rates are high.

Dosage: Aldara is applied 3 times a week and preferably prior to retiring to bed. The cream has to remain on the infected skin for 610 hours, after which time it is washed off. Treatment periods are usually 812 weeks.

Treatment efficacy: Aldara eradicates visible warts and minimizes recurrence since an immune response against the virus is provoked.

2. Actinic Keratosis

Actinic keratosis is a precancerous skin condition caused by long term exposure to ultraviolet (UV) radiation. Untreated, these rough, scaly patches of skin may progress to squamous cell carcinoma.

Dosage: Actinic Keratosis: Aldara cream is applied to the affected area 2 times per week, typically for 16 weeks. Even though the lesions may appear to clear before the end of therapy, the full treatment course should be completed.

Effectiveness: Aldara heightens the immune system's recognition and elimination of abnormal cells, significantly reducing the risk of cancer.

3. Superficial Basal Cell Carcinoma (sBCC)

Superficial basal cell carcinoma is a form of nonmelanoma skin cancer that, in most instances, can be treated without necessarily reverting to surgical intervention. One of the methods of treatment for those with superficial basal cell carcinoma and who prefer their treatment to be as noninvasive as possible includes the use of Aldara.

Dosage: The cream is applied 5 times a week for 6 weeks. It is also important that the patients apply the cream to the tumor site and wash it off after the recommended duration.

Effectiveness: Aldara is effective in shrinking small, superficial tumors, and thus may be used as an alternative treatment to surgical excision in certain cases.

OffLabel Uses

Off Label use of Aldara has been made in the treatment of molluscum contagiosum, cutaneous leishmaniasis, and even some cases of melanoma in situ. Even though these indications are not approved by the FDA, clinical evidence points to the immunostimulatory potential of Aldara in the treatment of various skin conditions.

CHAPTER TWO

Application and Usage

Correct application of Aldara is vital not only for effectiveness but also to minimize side effects arising from its use. It comes in the form of a cream, usually in small sachets or tubes.

Steps Involved in Application:

1. Cleanse the Affected Area: The affected area should be cleaned carefully with mild

soap and water before application, then patted dry.

2. Apply Thin Layer: Squeeze a small amount onto your fingertip and apply a thin layer to the affected area. Do not apply too much,

as this can make skin irritation more likely.

3. Wash Hands: After application, wash your hands to avoid accidental spreading to any other area.

4. Leave On the Skin: Leave the cream on the skin for

approximately 610 hours, which would again depend on the nature of the ailment. For better results, this cream is applied before retiring to bed.

5. Rinse Off: Wash the treated area after the time with soap and water.

Frequency of Application:

In cases of genital warts, Aldara is normally applied 3 times a week.

For actinic keratosis, it is used 2 times a week.

For superficial basal cell carcinoma, it is applied 5 times per week.

Duration:

The duration is different for all the conditions, but generally varies from 8 to 16 weeks.

Side Effects of Aldara

While Aldara is well tolerated, it does result in local skin reactions and systemic side effects. Generally, these reactions are mild but can sometimes be more severe, especially if the cream is misused or applied too much.

Common Side Effects:

Redness and Irritation: Mild to moderate redness, itching,

or burning at the application site may commonly occur. Flaking and Peeling: This can happen as the response of the immune system to the abnormal cells or viral infection. Swelling: There is a possibility of swelling around the area treated; this is more pronounced in areas like the face or genitals. Crusting or Scabbing: In the process of destruction of the abnormal cells, the area may form scabs or crusts; this is part of the normal healing process.

Ulceration and Erosion: Rarely, Aldara can lead to the ulceration of skin or heavy erosion, especially in cases where the application is made more than the prescribed frequency or for longer periods than recommended.

Flu Like Symptoms: Other systemic adverse effects reported by some patients include tiredness, fever, aching muscles, and headaches.

Infection: The immune response generated from using Aldara may lead to secondary infections in the place of its administration.

Managing Side Effects:

Decreased Frequency:

Application frequency may be reduced when severe reactions are noted, in order to give the skin time to recover.

Emollient Creams: Application of mild moisturizers or barrier creams facilitates healing of irritated skin.

Precautions and Contraindications

Aldara has to be used with added precaution in certain patients, whereas it is absolutely contraindicated in others.

Precautions:

Immune Disorders: Aldara is contraindicated in cases of autoimmune disorders, as it stimulates the immune system.

Pregnancy: Information regarding the safety of Aldara in pregnancy is lacking. This product is listed under Category C in pregnancy, meaning that risk cannot be ruled out. Physicians may wish to avoid use unless benefits outweigh potential risks.

Sun Exposure: It is best to avoid excessive exposure to the sun with the use of Aldara as the skin will be so much more sensitive and easily burned.

Contraindications:

Allergic Reactions: Aldara is not recommended for those who have, in the past, experienced allergic reactions from imiquimod or any of the ingredients in the cream.

Severe Inflammation: Aldara must not be used on an application site where inflammation and infection are serious until such time as the inflammation subsides.

Drug Interactions and Resistance

Unlike typical antiviral or anticancer drugs, Aldara does not attack pathogens or tumors directly; therefore, resistance is not considered a big problem with this medication. However, considering that the basis of its activity is the modulation of the immune response, there is some concern about its interaction with other immunomodulatory drugs or antiinflammatory agents.

Potential Interactions: Corticosteroids: Systemic or topical corticosteroids may reduce the effectiveness of Aldara by suppressing the immune response that Aldara induces.

Immunosuppressants: Those on immunosuppressive therapies for instance, because of an organ transplant cannot be fully treated with Aldara since the immune system is, for obvious reasons, suppressed.

Conclusion

Aldara, or Imiquimod, is a powerful drug that leverages the body's immune prowess to combat conditions of the skin, from HPVrelated genital warts to precancerous lesions and superficial basal cell carcinoma. Its possible use in altering the immune response makes it

It is a unique drug, useful in dermatology with a number of applications; hence, cautious application and monitoring are required to avoid any potential adverse effects.

By being aware of the action mechanisms underlying its formulation, its therapeutic uses, correct application methods, and adverse effects, both the patient and the professional can optimize this medication with minimal risk. In instances where skin conditions may require long term treatment or where treatments need to be conservative and less invasive, Aldara presents an excellent avenue for management.

THE END